Effective Acne Treatments That Work

"Best Whole Body Natural Acne Treatments That Get Results"

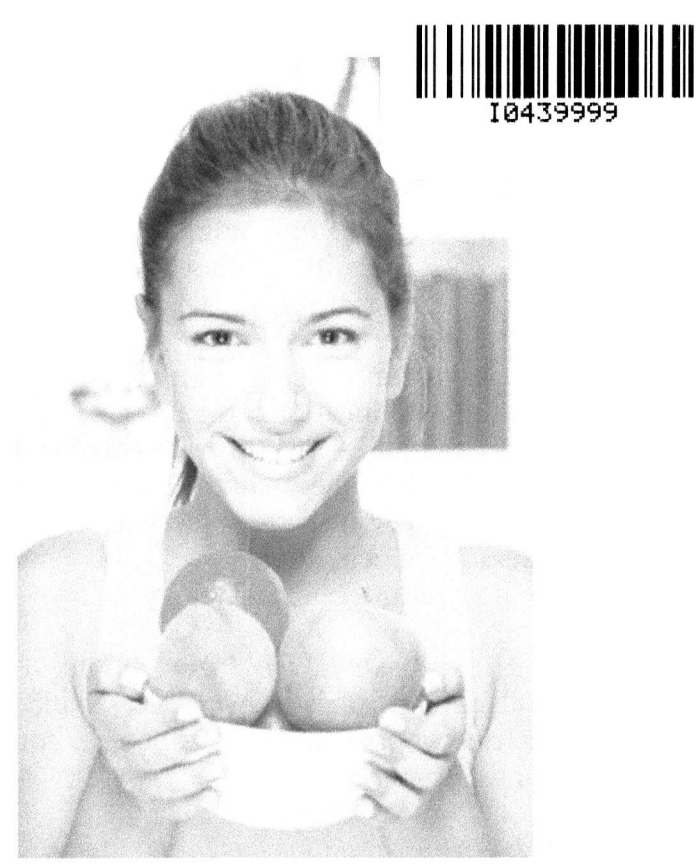

I0439999

By Rudy S. Silva, Natural Nutritionist

Dedication

This e-book is dedicated to Annie C. Campos who developed a severe case of acne in her early 20's and who started using the 12 step methods I have listed here.

Here persistence in using these processes has paid off for her and now has clearer skin. She still has to be careful with her diet, since she tends to breakout when eating the wrong foods.

In addition Annie Campos has worked hard to get this Acne e-book in Kindle form so that it would be available for you as a paperback book.

Table of Contents

Preface

Hi, my name is Rudy Silva and I'm a natural nutritional consultant who is concern with the pain and suffering that you experience in your life. I look for natural ways that you can relieve your pain and conditions so that you can minimize the use of drugs. In addition, I am an educator and I write to explain how your body works so that you get a good understanding of the condition you suffer from.

It is here in this book you find out what acne is all about and how you can deal with it in a natural and healing way. This report is not about creating a miracle, where you will eliminate acne in three days or less.

It is about applying known cleansing techniques and nutritional and herbal remedies that give you better health and better facial skin. The way you look and the way you think is a reflection of what it looks like inside your body. And, the way the inside of your body looks like is reflected on your face, physical appearance and your thoughts.

If you are serious and motivate about getting rid of acne, then this book will give you all the details you need to know to get a clear face. It's not easy to do, but it works. I cannot guarantee that next week you will be free of acne. The amount of work you put into clearing your acne will determine how quickly your face becomes blemish free.

If your acne is heredity, it is not true that you cannot do anything about it. If you know that other members of the family have had acne and previous generations also, then you are susceptible to acne. Knowing this, you can now arm yourself with some powerful nutritional and hygiene habits that will prevent acne from taking hold and remaining for what can seem like forever.

1: Acne Is A Disease

Acne is a disease called seborrhea or seborrheic dermatitis. It occurs when the sebaceous glands, under your skin, become contaminated with oily toxic matter, which contains,

- dirt
- dead skin
- excess sebum oil
- acid waste
- bacteria
- toxic matter

DHT

Under normal conditions the sebaceous glands release oil that comes up through your pores onto your skin surface. This release keeps your skin moist and lubricated for protection against the environment.

If the pores on your face are not open or plugged, this oil moves into your pores and cannot move out onto your skin. If this oil remains trapped, it can be come toxic. This results in the growth of a pimple that starts to increase in size and becomes more toxic as oil tries to reach the surface of your skin.

If pore walls burst under the skin, white blood cells move in to digest the collagen around the pores. When this happens, you will have scars on your face.
To avoid having scars, you need to start an acne-cleaning program, before you get acne or just as soon as you see acne coming so that your pimples and back heads don't get to the point where they get severely infected and burst.

Clearing Your Acne

Acne is a complex condition that involves many parts of the body even though it shows up only as eruptions on your face and elsewhere on your skin. It is a signal that you have problems inside your body caused by your diet, hormones, poor health, or stress. Acne is caused by the lifestyle you live.

To clear acne, it is not always possible to just do one thing and expect acne to go away. But it may be possible to just use a special cream and have your acne diminish or clear. It may go away by just doing one thing but don't expect it to. A facial cream, diet, herbal treatment, and colon cleanse alone may not be able to clear acne. A combination may or may not work.

For this reason I, have come up a facial acne cleansing technique and a twelve step acne clearing process so that you will have a better chance of clearing your acne.

For a beautiful Face

To have beautiful, soft, radiant skin you need to eat plenty of the right fresh fruits, vegetables and water. Water is critical because it moves toxins out of your body using the normal channels of elimination, rather than by using your skin. A word of Caution: Sudden face or body eruptions can indicate a potentially serious medical condition. If your blemishes look large and like welts, this could be caused by a serious medical condition and you would need to see your Doctor immediately.

Traditional Medical Acne Treatments

There is a traditional facial treatment that you can start with to give your facial skin some help as you pursue the other natural methods described in this book. This treatment will be described in the next chapters.

But here are some products you should know about and their effects on your skin.

Benzoyl peroxide for dark skinned – opens pores to kill bacteria

Antibiotics – erythromycin, tetracycline – kills bacteria everywhere it goes in your body and skin.

Retin A – helps to break open plugged pores, prevents new plugged pores, and helps to prevent scarring.

Topical steroid, cortisone derivative, drug

These drugs and many others have serious side effects that you will want to avoid. If you are dark skinned and are using Benzoyl Peroxide, you can end up spotting your face by changing your skin tone.

Most of these medications take three to ten weeks to provide results.

All of my recommendations use natural remedies for eliminating acne, except for the main acne facial treatment, which uses drugstore creams or creams that you can buy on the internet.

An Acne Face Cream That Helps Acne

Here is a natural cream created by Doug Cooper from the Bay Area, in California. Doug is an ordinary man who has a deep sincere motivation to help people who have body pain and skin conditions.

His acne cream is called Scotty's Acne cream. It contains the entire spectrums of minerals, trace minerals, and specific oil extracts that promoted tissue rebuilding, conditioning, and recovery. To have good skin you need to concentrate on getting more minerals into your body and skin. Your health is in the minerals.

This cream formulation was made the way it should be since,

- It contained all natural ingredients
- It contained natural oils that rejuvenate the skin
- It contain minerals that help to reduce inflammation and rebuild the cell structure
- It contain nutrients that promoted skin regeneration and healing

Doug's cream is excellent for acne. You can use other creams that you have found, but make sure the ingredients are natural.

2: Parts of the body That Affect Acne

To clear your acne permanently, you need to get to the cause. There can be one or many causes. These causes can depend on your genetics, your emotional state, and diet history.

Yes, you can work on your face with various creams, topological drugs, or washes. This will get you some relief and may even eliminate your acne. But sometimes, if the cause of acne is not eliminated, then pimples will keep coming back.

The actual cause of acne comes from internal organs or body systems that are overloaded and cannot correctly process toxins and hormones. The result is that these toxins and hormones accumulate or create accumulations in your skin pores and cause acne.

What is acne?

"Acne is a skin condition that frequently shows up on the face or other skin surfaces as an inflamed area called a pimple or blemish that is filled with bacteria, oil, dead skin cells, and other toxic material." As this inflamed area progresses, it can continue to grow until it burst or you burst it. Scaring can result if you scratch it, pick at it, or prevent it from healing on its own.

Where do these bacteria, fungus, oils and toxic matters come from and how can you stop it from forming?

Let's first look at how toxic matter is created and handled by the body. The body has 6 channels of elimination and detoxification. Each channel is responsible for eliminating or detoxifying toxic material that can harm the inside and outside of your body. These channels are,

- The colon
- The kidney
- The lungs
- The lymphatic system
- The skin
- Liver

The Colon

The colon is where most illnesses, body ills or symptoms start and this includes your acne. These illnesses result from eating food that is not beneficial for your body.

Toxins that originate and are created in the colon are acid waste. This acid waste, when it gets into your blood and skin causes inflammation. This is the waste that you need to make sure does not get into your blood and come out of your face.

If acid waste does get into your blood, which some will, you want to have an excess of minerals in your body to neutralize this waste. This is why having an alkaline body and not an acid body is critical for eliminating acne. So, getting a lot of minerals into your body will help you turn your acid body into an alkaline body.

The first thing you want to know about your colon is whether you are constipated. When you are constipated, the colon will allow more acid waste to get into your blood.

What does constipation have to do with acne?

Most people are constipated. It is typical for people to go 2-3 days without a bowel movement. Some doctors say it's ok or normal for this to happen. It's not ok. If you want to become seriously ill in the future and you want to struggle with acne for a long time than it might be ok. Fecal matter that stays in your colon more than normal,

- affects the health of your colon
- causes colon wall inflammation
- decays and become toxic
- hardens
- interferes with absorption of nutrients
- kills good bacteria that keeps you healthy
- promotes multiplication of bad bacteria
- sticks to your colon walls
- weakens your colon walls
- moves slowly in the colon
- becomes stagnant and doesn't move for days
- becomes difficult in coming out
- takes a long time to come out

So what can you do about constipation? You will find out what to do about constipation in step 3.

The kidney

The purpose of the two kidneys is to filter the water in the blood as the blood passes through the kidneys. About 4 gallons of water are filtered every day, but only around 3 pints are pulled out as urine.

Alcohol and sugar are the most damaging to the kidneys, since they kill kidney cells and weaken kidney function.

Water is the major way the body keeps toxins from accumulating in your body and skin. You need to drink plenty of clean water daily, so your kidneys can remove toxins and excess nutrients, vitamins, and minerals from your blood.

When you drink plenty of water, the skin does not have to act as a water filter to filter out excess waste from the blood, since it is been filter and excreted as urine, by your kidney.

Water also is needed to keep your skin moist. Water in the skin layers helps to protect the skin from bacteria and toxins that try to pass into your skin.

The more fresh juices you drink and the more fruit or vegetables you eat, the less water you need to drink. All juices contain plenty of distilled water, which contributes to your daily water requirement.

Drinking sodas and other drinks that have sugar cannot be counted as water.

The Lungs

You have two large sacs that are called lungs. As you breathe in air, the lungs pull oxygen out of the air. This oxygen is captured by your blood, routed to your liver, moved into your heart, and then moved into all parts of your body.

As you breathe out, waste and carbon dioxide are routed to your lung by your blood and pushed out through your mouth.

Your cells use oxygen to create energy for you to live by. You need energy for every movement your body does. Oxygen is also used to neutralize waste and pathogen. The more acid waste and pathogens you have in your body, the more oxygen is used up to neutralize them. This means you will have less oxygen for other body functions.

If the other elimination channels are weak and overloaded, the lungs will also become overloaded trying to get rid of waste the other channels cannot get rid of.

The result of weak lungs is that more waste stays in the body, making your body more acidic and susceptible to disease and infections. This waste and toxins need to be eliminated and that is where your skin comes in. Your skin has a great surface area, so this is where a lot of toxins are eliminated. If you have a lot of body odor, these are toxins being eliminated.

Lymphatic System

The lymphatic system is part of your immune system. It consists of a series of tubes, large and small, that cover your entire body. Through these tubes flow whitish liquid called lymph. Since this system does not have a pump, like your heart, the lymph is pushed through the tubes by your body's movement, such as exercise, walking, or jumping.

Lymph liquid surrounds all of your body cells and is responsible for bringing nutrients to your cells from your blood. It is moves toxins that come out of your cells into the lymphatic tubes, through the lymph nodes and into the blood stream.

Toxins and pathogens that are in your lymph liquid are moved into lymph nodes. In the lymph nodes, this toxic matter is neutralized into harmless chemicals and then moved into the blood and eliminated through the other channels of elimination.

The lymph liquid is composed of electrolyte minerals such as sodium, potassium, calcium, phosphorus, and chloride. So, strong lymph liquid is built when you eat fruits and vegetables.

When the lymph nodes become overwhelmed with toxic waste from the cells, they become inflamed and cannot keep your body free of toxic matter. Excess toxic waste accumulates in your lymph liquid when your body does not have enough electrolyte minerals to neutralize this toxic acidic waste. Now, your body is considered acidic and will have a difficult time fighting infections, such as acne.

The skin

The skin is the largest of the elimination channels. Through the skin, toxins are eliminated, which are brought to the skin surface from the blood. When the regular elimination channels are sluggish or partial plugged up, such as your colon by being constipated, toxins do not move out through your stools. In fact, toxins that accumulate in your colon tend to move into your blood. Once in your blood, they move into your liver for detoxification.

If you are frequently constipated, than your liver will be overworked and unable to detoxify all of your colon toxins. The liver will store a lot of toxins in its own tissue and elsewhere in your body's tissues, joints, organs, cells and skin.

But when you have excessive toxins, they moved to the skin surface, through your blood, where they enter your hair pores – follicles – and try to move to the skin surface. Body odor is a result of toxins coming out through your skin that should be moving out through the other elimination channels.

If your skin, throughout your body, is clean and its pores are open and unclogged, toxins will move out through the pores without creating pimples or eruptions. The skin normally moves 1-2 pounds of toxins out of your skin daily.

You can tell when your pores are open. You sweat freely during exercise. If you do not sweat much during hot weather or during exercise, then some of your skin pores might be plugged.

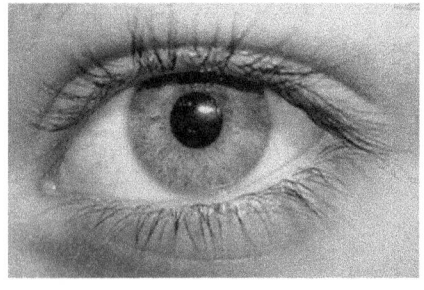

How can you tell if your skin is not breathing and working correctly? You can do this by looking into your eye or having someone else do it using a 10x magnifying glass. Look at the outer edge of your iris and if it is clear with no visible dark ring around it, then you have good skin function.

If your iris has a dark band or ring around it, it indicates that your skin is somewhat inactive and does not allow toxins to readily move out to your skin's surface. The skin needs to be activated so that it can work better in eliminating toxins.

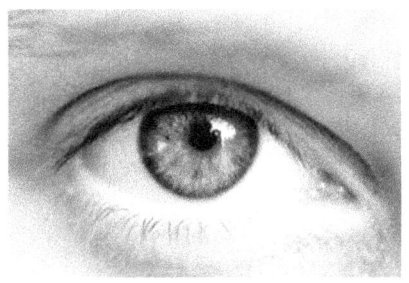 When you see the dark band around your iris, the darker and wider it appears the more severe your skin condition. The smaller and lighter it is the less severe is your skin inactivity.

This inspection of your iris just gives you some information on the health of your skin. To keep your skin active and serving as a good channel of elimination you need to brush your skin daily before you shower or during your shower.

Doing a colon cleanse helps to give your skin a rest and a chance to increase its function. If you can eliminate more toxins from your body through a body cleanse the less your skin has to work. In a future chapter I show you how you can eat, so that every day you are cleansing your body.

In her book, Detox For Life, 2002, Loree Taylor Jordan, C.C.H., I.D. says,

"One of greatest gifts of health that you can give yourself is the gift of skin brushing. Dry skin brushing is one of the finest of all baths. No soap can wash the skin as clean as the new skin you have under the old. You make new skin on the body every 24 hours. The skin will only be as clean as the bloodstream. Dry skin brushing removes the top layer. This helps to eliminate uric acid crystals catarrh, and various other acids in the body. The skin should eliminate 2 pounds of waste acids daily."

Liver

The liver is responsible for detoxifying all your body's blood as it comes from the colon, lungs, and lymphatic system. Once detoxified, this blood moves into your entire body to provide your cells with oxygen and digested nutrients.

Because you drink, eat and breathe in so many toxins, the liver has a hard time neutralizing the toxins coming from the colon. If you are constipated, this puts an extreme toxic load on the liver, which eventually leads to the excretion of these toxins through your skin and face.

All cellular wastes and excess hormones are routed to the liver through your lymphatic system. Once in the liver, the liver starts the detoxifying process. If the liver is overloaded with toxins, it will start to store these toxins in its own cells, in the cells of your organs, in your joints, in your skin, or any other place that it can find.

Hormones such as androgens that are not neutralized can get back into the blood and move into the cells, where they pile up and cause an over production of sebum that will flow into your hair follicle.

If you are a typical eater, then most likely you have been surviving on junk food. The quantity of toxic chemicals and non-food additives that are in the food you eat accumulates in your colon, your liver, your blood, and in your face as toxins. These toxins need to be neutralized and eliminated through various organs. If you are constantly supplying toxins to your body, these organs will get overloaded.

All junk food and processed food is detrimental to your health and to your face or skin. Once you stop punishing yourself and forcing your body to process toxic food products, you will have a chance of clearing your colon, liver, blood and the blemished conditions of your face.

What other body conditions contribute to toxic or acid waste?

There are three other areas that you need to know about that contribute to acid waste. If these areas are not working properly, then acid waste is created.

- Mental attitude
- Stomach acid

- Pancreatic digestive enzymes

Acne is an expression of toxins in your body that are not being released through normal channels of elimination. If these toxins are not eliminated normally then they will come out through your skin. Since mental attitude and thoughts cannot be separate from the body, thoughts and feelings are also being expressed as acne.

Negative thoughts and feeling are known to produce chemicals that are toxic acids. Just like toxic acids created in the colon or by food, your toxic thoughts need to be eliminated through the five elimination channels.

Acne can be an expression of low esteem. So you create a condition on your face that coincides with your feelings. Acne gives you a reason not like yourself or your life because your face is filled with eruptions that are unsightly. The way you feel inside is always expressed by the way you look outside.

Acne can also be related to the emotion of fear or anxiety. It can also be an expression of holding onto old junkie or unpleasant memories. It's a way of holding on to and burying the junkie or toxic memory into your face. It is these memories that are trying to surface and face you straight on, but you may not be ready to know what these traumatic memories are and far less ready to deal with them.

Stomach Acid

Your stomach uses Hydrochloric acid (HCl) to break down protein. It also has many other functions, such as,

- killing pathogens and microbes
- controlling the adsorption of B12
- controlling the adsorption of iron calcium zinc, copper, magnesium and most B-complex vitamins
- controlling the adsorption of vitamin C
- creating indigestion

- preventing constipation

When you have low levels of HCl, stomach acid, chances are that you will be susceptible to getting acne. Low levels of HCL can come from taking drugs or using acid reflux products. These products decrease your HCL levels so that you will not suffer from high stomach acid levels.

Pancreatic Digestive Enzymes

When the food you eat passes the stomach and enters the small intestine, the pancreas releases digestive enzymes and bicarbonate to help complete the digestive process.

The bicarbonate helps to reduce the acid strength of the food coming from your stomach. The digestive enzymes digest carbohydrates, fats, and protein that were not digested in the stomach.

When the pancreas loses its efficiency and starts to release less digestive enzymes, less food is properly digested, as it should be. This results in more undigested food reaching the colon. When this happens, the undigested food, if it stays to long in the colon, becomes a source of rotting matter and toxic material.

A healthy pancreas, which provides the necessary digestive juices to digest the food you eat, is needed for healthy skin and for eliminating acne and skin sores, and eruptions.

3: Main Acne Facial Cleansing

Use this facial cleansing method in conjunction with those methods that call for internal cleansing and taking specific supplements to clean up your internal organs.

By combining both methods, you are attacking your acne from the inside, which gives you long term acne curing and from the outside, which gives you relief and curing of your present acne.

In this method, you will be working directly on your skin to start healing the facial blemishes that you now have. Follow the instructions carefully so that you get the best results. If you start to deviate from the instructions you go against a time tested method that has produced excellent results for others.

An outline of the Acne Facial Cleansing Method

Here is the outline of this facial process that you need to follow and approximately what it will cost. Since this program is for 4 – 7 weeks you may have to buy larger units. These prices will change as time passes.

Using Salicylic Acid ....$12.00 plus shipping
Using Glycolic Acid..............$25.50 plus shipping
Using Benzoyl peroxide ......$15.00 or $20.00 plus shipping
Using a Moisturizer.............$15.00 plus shipping
Night Cream ....$16.00 plus shipping

You will need to use these different cleansing methods at the same time. Doing them separate has been found not to be effective in getting rid of acne.

Using Salicylic Acid

The first step is to use salicylic acid. When you use salicylic acid on your face, it serves to remove dead skin cells, and the dead cells that combine with your sebum to plug up your pores at the surface of your skin. It also helps reduce the bad bacteria that can accumulate on the surface of your skin.

Salicylic acid also provides an anti-inflammatory benefit by reducing the inflammation around your pores. This helps to open these pores slightly and allows salicylic acid to move deeper into the pores to clean them out.

Buy a 2 % salicylic acid and no less. You can go to the internet and get this acid or go to your favorite drug store and ask for it. This product comes in pads or gel.

Applying the salicylic acid

This how you apply salicylic acid and you will do this for 6 weeks twice a day – first thing in the morning and the last thing at night.

If you have acne in different parts of your face or body start with one area then go to the next area.

First, you splash warm water onto your face. Put about the size of a dime or more of salicylic acid on your hand.

Mix the a few drops of distilled water into salicylic acid. Make sure the two are mixed well. This dilutes the salicylic acid.

In a circular movement, rub the salicylic acid and water mixture into the area that is covered with acne.

Now, go to the next area that has acne, wet that area with water, then rub in the salicylic acid like before.

Leave the salicylic acid on your face for about 5 minutes or for the time as instruction on the salicylic package.

Using Glycolic Acid

To unplug and dissolve the follicles of dead cells and sebum, which occur deep into the follicles, you need to use glycolic acid. It is this trapped mixture of dead cells and sebum that plug up the follicles that lead to infected pimples.

Use an 8-10% glycolic acid with no other active additives. Here two products you can use. You may find a pad or a gel product.

Glycolic acid is used immediately after you use salicylic acid and you use it in just the same way. Let it stay on your skin for 3-5 minutes. Then, rinse it off with warm water and go take a shower, if it is morning.

Use Glycolic acid only once a day and in the morning.

Completing Two Steps in the Facial Cleaning

Now that you have done the Salicylic and Glycolic acid cleansing, you have accomplished:

Cleansing your face of bacteria that can continue flowing into pores and creating new infections on your face

Removing many of the plugs made of up of dead cells and sebum that form at the opening of your pores.

Removing the dead cells and excess oil across your skin to exposed new skin and to active the healing process

Using Benzoyl Peroxide (BP)

Now, for the third step in this facial process, you will use Benzoyl Peroxide or BP. Using BP will stabilize your face more, since the first steps still leave the pores on your face inflamed, with pus, bacteria and excess sebum.

This pus and other material are way down into your pores or follicles, where it is hard to get to. If this pus is not removed it will just continue to create the acne you are trying to get rid of.

Using BP allows you to move oxygen deep into your pores where it acts as an antibacterial application preventing bacteria buildup and killing any bacteria embedded deep into the pores.

Here's how to use BP. First buy a 10% solution of benzoyl peroxide. You may need to go to the internet to buy it, if you can't find it at your drug store.

Use BP in the evening after you use Salicylic Acid. Here's how to start.

Store your BP in the refrigerator and allow it to cool before You use it.

Freeze some distilled water into ice cubes. Take an ice cube and rub it across your acne infected area. Just get your skin cold and wet, but don't leave the ice cube to long on your face otherwise you can freeze your skin.

Place a few drops of BP on your palm of your hand or on a cold dish that was in the refrigerator. If you use your palm, cool it down with an ice cube and then put a few drop of BP onto it.

Prepare and apply the BP just like you did with Salicylic acid. Add a drop of water to BP, mix it, and then rub it in a circular motion onto the infected area. If you already have water in your hand, mix that with your BP.

After you have applied the BP, place cold packs from the refrigerator onto your infected area. If you are working with two infected areas, then you need to apply a cold pack to each one. Get a thin cloth or paper towel to place between the cold pack and your facial skin to prevent burning your skin from the cold pack. If your skin gets to cold, use a thicker cloth.

Leave this cold pack on for 8-11 minutes. You may have to be in a lying position to keep the cold packs in position.

After the 8- 11 minute cold pack, wipe your face off with some clean cloth and leave the BP residue on your face overnight.

There you are the third step in the facial cleansing process.

Now, if after you using BP you sense an excessive burning or itching, you can alternate the use of BP with Glycolic acid every other day. But use the Glycolic acid just as describe for the BP, ice and everything else.

If you just feel some tingling and no uncomfortable burning on your face, after BP, then you can use it every day.

These three steps should get rid of your acne in 4- 7 weeks or less.

Using a Moisturizer

Now, for the final easy step, you need to use a moisturizer everyday after you have cleansed your skin in the morning with salicylic and glycolic acid.

The moisturizer will help to keep your skin healthy looking and resistant to the start of new acne.

Here's the type of moisturizer you need to use:

- Oil free
- Moisturizer with sun block of 15 or higher

Use the moisturizer 2-3 times a day, if you feel your skin drying out or if you are in the sun for a long period. You may want to renew your moisturizer, on your face, to get more sun block onto your skin.

If you can find a cream that is all natural with sun block then buy it and use it.

Partially Natural Moisturizer with Sun block

After Your 6 Weeks Program and No Acne

Once you have gotten rid of your acne, now you need to keep a facial cleansing program that will maintain your clear skin.

First, continue using the moisturized mentioned above.

Second, use a cleansing cream that has glycolic acid, two to three times a week, before you put your moisturizer on. Rub this cream into the area that was infected with acne. Then put on your moisturizing cream.

Every night just before bedtime, use a night cream that has vitamin C ester, Tocotrienols, and Alpha Lipoic Acid. Tocotrienols are members of the vitamin E family. Some times you can find this cream with all three ingredients or as separate creams.

Again go to the internet to find your natural products, since many of the normal products have so many petroleum ingredients and other chemicals that are not good for your skin. Shop carefully for full natural products and treat your skin right.

There you have it, a facial cleansing process that will eliminate acne and a simple program to use to keep your skin healthy and free of future acne breakouts.

Use these special secret techniques and you will be free of acne before you know it.

4: Second Acne Facial Cleansing

An Acne Remedy When Your Kidney is Weak

First, you will have acne, if your kidney is unable to detoxify toxins. These toxins will move into your skin and combined with other matter to cause pimples, if you do keep your face skin clean and working properly.

So, the first thing you need to do is keep your face clean. Here's how to do it.

1. Buy some Bragg's Apple Cider Vinegar
2. Buy a complexion brush or some large soft cotton balls (or you can use your clean finger tips)
3. Jojoba oil with 10% or so of tree tea oil, or one bottle of each oil and mix them

Mixing the Apple Cider Vinegar

Mix apple cider vinegar with warm distilled water. Heat the distilled water to warm using only a glass or ceramic pot.

To start with, use 10 parts water to 1 part apple cider vinegar. If your skin is not real sensitive you can use a stronger mixture, all the way to a 50:50 mixture. That is, mix ½ apple cider vinegar to ½ distilled warm water.

Cleaning Your Face

First wash your face with room temperature water but do not use soap. You don't need to dry your face after washing.

Now, pour a little apple cider vinegar mixture onto your

fingers and massage it onto your face for a few minutes.

Now, dip the complexion brush or cotton pads into the apple cider vinegar mixture and softly scrub your face to remove dirt and dead skin. The cotton pad will absorb a lot of liquid, so you want to carefully not to drip all over your face and counter. You may want to experiment with a facial sponge or another type of material.

I found it easier to dip my fingers in the cider mixture and then rub it on my face. Just make sure you clean your hands with a good natural soap.

When scrubbing your face with this mixture be careful not to get it into your eyes. If you need to scrub your forehead, lean your head down and do not soak the cotton balls since the mixture will drip all over your face. Just go slow until you see how to us this mixture.

The apple cider vinegar will leave your skin acidic and this is the normal pH balance for your skin. An acid skin will prevent bacteria and other pathogen from getting past your skin barrier. An alkaline skin will breed bacteria.

Do this skin cleansing, with the apple cider vinegar, three times a day.

After brushing your skin, rinse your face once with warm water, and then pat your face dry. For those places on your face that become dry, use Jojoba oil mixed with tree tea oil.

After I use the 50:50 cider mixtures, my face is dry after about 5-7 minutes. My skin feels tight and a little stingy. So I put about ½ dropper of jojoba and tree tea oil onto my hands and rub it all over my face.

Go here to read more about how jojoba and tree tea oil are good for skin conditions.

Look on the internet to get a jojoba and tree tea mixture.

Or you can go to your health store and buy bottle jojoba oil and a bottle of tree tea oil. This is what I did. Then I mixed the two by adding 1 part of tree tea oil to 9 parts jojoba oil. When mixing these oils, I just eyeballed the quantities to mix.

You can buy a clean dropper bottle at the health food store so you can combine the jojoba and tree tea oil.

Kidney cleanse

Now, here is the next thing you need to do. You need to cleanse your kidney. If you have a good functioning kidney, it will remove toxic material out of your blood and move it out your urine.

If your kidneys are weak, it can't remove all of the toxic material out of your blood so it stays in the blood and gets routed to your skin to be excreted.

So here what you need to do. Buy Dr. Schulze kidney-cleansing kit. Look for it on the internet.

The information on how to do this kidney cleanse is in Dr. Schulze's kidney kit. Buy his 5-Day Detox - Kidney Program. It contains,
- K-B Formula
- K-B Tea
- Detox Formula

This kidney kit, which uses herbs, will help you flush and detoxify your kidneys and bladder.

Some acne or certain skin conditions are really difficult to eliminate. Skin conditions are normally a result of weak internal elimination organs. This causes these organs to route toxins, that they would normal eliminate, to the skin for elimination.

If you have acne or other skin condition, it is a reflection of the lifestyle and food that you have been eating all of your life. Yes there are other people who have the same lifestyle and eating habits that you have and they don't get acne.

People, who have a poor lifestyle and don't have acne, have some other health issues that are either external of internal. At some point in their life these issue can become serious.

Toxins that have to be eliminated from the body and are not eliminated through the normal elimination channels will go to the weakest part of the body for elimination or for storage.

This part of the body is different for each person. Some people have a weakness in the skin, some in their heart, and some in their liver and so on.

5: The Twelve Step Acne Program

What I am about to tell you is how you can get your face clear of acne. I know there is lot of claims that you can only do it with creams or facial products. Yes, you will get some relief and in some cases you will eliminate your acne.

For those that need more than a special cream like Scotty's then you need to work harder to get rid of acne. Since acne is a condition that is cause from within your body and shows its self on your skin, you need to,

- attack the problem from inside your body
- attack the problem from outside your body

If your acne is not too severe, all you might need is a good cream and need only to follow a few steps in my 12 step program to get you past the periods where your acne is active.

If your acne is more severe, than you may have to follow my 12-step program, since acne is an expression of your whole body system and is a reflection of what is going on inside your mind, cell structure and internal organs.

You will be using Scotty's cream or some other natural acne cream to help repair, relieve, and rejuvenate your skin. You may also need to do the facial cleansing mentioned earlier.

Here is where you can find Scotty's,

http://www.bestgameproducts.com/products/?pid=1 2

If this link is no longer active, go to Google and just search for

Scotty's Acne Cream.

Then you will be following an internal program to reduce the amount of toxins in your body.

Acne is an excessive toxic and/or hormonal condition within your body, which the internal elimination organs are unable to eliminate. So your toxins are moved into your blood and excreted through your skin. It is an automatic survival mechanism your body initiates in an effort to protect the insides of your body – cells, liquid, blood, organs, tissue and so on.

Starting the 12 Steps

Following this program will provide you with a nutritional program that can become part of your lifestyle that will give you tremendous health benefits in the future.

There are 12 areas that you need to look at,

- Keeping your face clean
- Using Scotty's acne face cream
- Relieving your constipation and through the three day liquid fast
- Making changes to your diet
- Taking the Vitamins you need
- Taking the Minerals you should be
- Using special supplements
- Drinking Herbal mixture
- Drinking special detoxifying drinks
- Brushing your skin
- Changing your attitude

6: Step 1 - Keeping your face clean

If you use facial cosmetics, you need to stop. Some cosmetic irritate the skin and can cause acne by plugging up the pores on your face. The cosmetics chemicals that can cause you the most irritation and pore inflammation are:

- mineral oil
- lanolin
- parabens
- propylene glycol

Look at the label of the cosmetics you use. You will find that many cosmetics, soaps, and sunscreens contain these and harmful chemicals.

You need to get a clean face to start this program.

Find a water base make up, not an oil base one that does not irritate your face and use it sparingly.

When you wash your face don't use any commercial soaps, since they are filled with chemicals that will irritate and worsen your acne condition. And, don't wash your face too often as this will dry your skin of your natural protective oil. Also, don't keep touching your face, since you spread or add bacteria to it.

To wash your face use only Castile hand or liquid soap or Pure Glycerin hand soap

You can pat your face with a clean hot face towel to bring circulation to your face and to help open and move the toxic material, in the pimple, to the surface. Do not scrub hard to burst a pimple but just scrub lightly to burst a pimple when it is ready to open.

Use the hot towel application only 2-3 times per week.

When a pimple is open do not continue to rub or scrub it. In fact, do not pick or scratch an open pimple, since this could create other sores or leave scars that are difficult to remove. Just washing your face with clean soap will keep your face free of toxic matter.

Keep in mind that whatever you put on your skin will move into your skin and into your bloodstream.

Most commercial creams, lotions, and soaps are filled with all kinds of chemicals that are toxic to your body. By using them, you are making your liver work harder. A good working liver is a good defense against acne.

During the day or night avoid resting your cheeks or chin on your hand(s) or arm(s). This can irritate your face and cause acne to breakout. When you sleep, try to sleep on your back and not with your face or the side of your face on or into your pillow. Also be carefully about the soaps you use to wash your sheets. They retain the soap chemicals and these can irritate your facial skin.

Herbal face wash

After you wash your face with soap, you can use an herbal tea wash, if you like. This is a very simple thing to do and requires only two to three herbs. This herbal tea wash will have a healing and soothing effect on the open acne sores.

Here's what to do,

Add one tablespoon of Yarrow Root and ginger root into one cup of water. Boil the water then let the tea sit 10 -15 minutes off the heater plate. Strain the tea, and after it cools down, wash your face with it. Use it 3-4 times a day, if you like. Here are some other herbs you can use and what their activities are on your skin.

Fennel - has oleic acid, linolenic acid with high levels of tocopherols, flavonoids, protein, sugars, vitamins, calcium and potassium. It is has antibacterial and cytotoxic properties.

Chamomile - contains fatty acids, amino acids, and choline. It has a sedative and emollient effect and normalizes rough skin. It has bacterial and fungicidal properties.

Basil – has a high concentration of vitamin A and C. Used as an antiwormal and insect repellent.

Hyssop - can be used for treating skin irritations, burns, or psoriasis.

Sage - is used as a skin purifier. It is for greasy skin and provides fragrance. It has microbial action.

Yarrow - has a soothing effect on the skin and is anti inflammatory and non phototoxic.

Burdock Root – provides skin circulation

Chaparral – increases the circulation of your skin.

Comfrey leaves – give relief to an irritated skin.

Eucalyptus – heals skin irritation. It can help in regulating sebum production and cleans scalp and pores. It is also an anti-inflammatory.

Nettles or Stinging Nettles – cleans and stimulates the scalp

Ginger - contain lecithin, fatty acids protein, vitamins, and minerals. It is a stimulant for the vascular system and can provide some blood circulation activity in your skin.

Ginseng - contains many different chemicals that the body needs. It has sterols, pectin, vitamin B12 nicotinic acid, pantothenic acid, biotin, and choline minerals like zinc, copper, manganese, calcium, and iron and many more minerals.

MSM

When you make your facial teas, add MSM to the tea. MSM is great for your skin and will act as a delivery system for the herbs by moving them into your skin and pores. Add two MSM torpedoes, 2000mg, to your tea after it has cooled down. When you rinse your face with this tea, leave it on your face until it dries. This gives the herbs time to work on your skin. Rinse your face three times with this herbal tea.

7: Step 2 - Using Scotty's Acne Face Cream

After you have washed your face and used the herbal tea, use an applicator to dip into Scotty's face cream, but don't use your fingers. Place the cream on your face and spread it all around. Massage the cream into your face gently, so the skin absorbs the oils in this cream.

These oils will seal the pores and hold the natural moisture of the skin and enhance the curing effects of the cream.

You can use the cream 2-3 times a day. It is best to use it after you have cleaned your face in the morning and right before you go to bed. You can also use it at noon time.

You can use Scotty's' cream under your makeup or over your makeup. It will work either way. However, it will work better on a clean face.

You will notice that when you apply the cream it will tingle in areas without sores and may sting in areas of open sores. This will pass and as it does, it should reduce the itchiness of any sores.

Scotty's cream has allantoin, which will help to clear acne sores. The oils, vitamin A and E, and minerals in Scotty's will help to feed rebuild, and rejuvenate your skin. The minerals also help to neutralize the toxic acids that has contaminated and inflamed the pores on your face.

During cleansing and fasting, more acid waste may come out of your pores. This is why Scotty's cream will help you to reduce the inflammation and the spread of your acne.

Tree Tea Oil

To make Scotty's cream even more powerful, you can add 5-10 drops of pure tree tea oil to a two-ounce container. You can experiment with the amount to add. You may want to add more drops to provide more tea tree oil for your face. But, do not use more than 15 drops.

Tree tea oil has been found to be effective in various skin disorders. It acts as an antiseptic, antifungal, and antibacterial. This oil helps to bring oxygen to the skin cells, which kills bacteria and fungus and helps to repair damaged skin caused by acne.

Borage Oil

There is one more thing that you can add to Scotty's face cream that will boost its acne clearing power. This is borage oil. Borage oil contains EPA and DHA, which helps to control excessive hormones that cause the over production of sebum.

It is the adrenal glands that produce streams of androgens during puberty. These large quantities of androgens help to activate bone growth and assist in bringing forth sexual maturity.

A side effect of these androgens is the release of excess oil from the oil glands near your follicles. This excess oil gives rise to

- black heads
- white heads
- pimples
- cysts

So here's what you can do to make Scotty's face cream even more effective,

Mix one or two capsules of Borage oil into the Scotty's cream

Do this by cutting the tip off of the Borage oil soft gel and squeeze the oil into the cream

There is a new form of EPA and DHA that is available in a product called Neptune Krill Oil (NKO)

Neptune Krill Oil (NKO)

NKO is the new EPA and DHA product, which maybe better to use than Borage Oil. NKO has the omega-3, EPA and DHA in the phospholipid form, which is easier for your cells to absorb compared with Borage oil. Borage oil contains the omega-3, EPA, and DHA in triglyceride form, which is more difficult for cells to absorb.

In addition, to putting NKO in Scotty's cream you can also take it as a supplement and get it working inside your body.

One other good property of NKO is that is does not have to be refrigerated like Borage does. It can be kept in a cool place in your cabinets. However, it does cost more than Borage oil.

Word of Caution: As with all creams and oils, if you get any rash or skin reactions when using them, discontinue their use.

8: Step 3 – Three Day Juice Colon Cleanse

Now, you are ready to get your bowels moving regular. If you eat 3 meals each day, you should have 2 bowel movements a day. If you only have one, then you are short 1 bowel movement.

Normally, if you have 3 full meals a day, you should have 3 bowel movements a day.

Don't be fooled by anyone that says one bowel movement in one or two days is ok. This is not true.

If you want to learn how to keep regular using natural remedies, than you can check out my e-book called,

"Constipation Natural Cures." Look for it on Google Search

So let's get started.

To get your bowels moving like they should, you need to, clean out what is in your colon right now. So the first day is for cleaning out your colon. The next two days is for cleaning the colon and to detoxify the body.

Doing a fast of a minimum of three days is the best way to start cleaning out the colon, to detoxify the blood, and rejuvenate your body. Just doing a fast for three days is not a cure all and it will require more work on your part by starting to eat more natural foods.

I consider this a mini-fruit juice fast. This is to start your body detoxifying. You can do this juice fast once a month for 2-3 days but leave out the prune juice and just drink the juices for

2-3 days. This gives your stomach, small and large intestine and liver a rest and a chance to rejuvenate.

This three day colon cleansing is outline in my "Colon and Blood Cleansing Diet."

In her extensive book, Cooking For Healthy Healing, 1991, Linda Rector-page, N.D., Ph.D., talks about what a fast does, "Fasting works by self-digestion. During a cleanse, the body in its infinite wisdom, will decompose and burn only the substances and tissue that are damaged, diseased, or unneeded, such as abscesses, tumors, excess fat deposits, and congestive wastes. Even a relatively short fast can accelerate elimination from the liver, kidneys, lungs and skin, often causing dramatic changes as masses of accumulated waste is expelled. Live foods and juices can literally pick up dead matter from the body and carry it away."

Day before the fast

The day before the fast, eat a large salad and two apples. This will give you plenty of fiber to scrub the walls of your colon as you move fecal matter out of your colon the following day.

First day of colon cleanse

Do this cleanse on a Saturday, Sunday or any other day that you don't have to go anywhere. You will be going to the bathroom all day and at times you need to be there quick.

Buy the following items.

- Organic apple juice – one gallon
- Organic apples – 6 for one day
- Organic prune juice – one quart
- When you first wake up in the morning, drink,
- 8 oz of prune juice
- 10 minutes later drink another 8oz of prune juice
- 10 minutes later again drink another 8 oz of prune juice

- wait 20 minutes than drink 8 oz of apple juice
- wait 30 minutes than drink another 8 oz of apple juice

If you haven't sped to the bathroom yet, you will in a little while.

Now you will be drink 8 oz of apple juice every hour until the end of the day. You can stop drinking apple juice around 5pm.

During the day you can eat three apples in the morning and 3 apples in the evening.

This process will clean out any fecal matter that has been sitting your colon for days and gets you ready for the next step.

Second way to start the colon cleanse

Another way to start a colon cleanse is to use a product that is called "Oxy-Powder." This product is in capsules and is used to 30 days. Simply by taking capsules everyday, you will clean out your colon and any build up along your colon walls.

This is a very effective product and will send you to the bathroom frequently as it clean out your colon. Start this cleanse on a Saturday so you can have Saturday and Sunday free to start cleaning out your colon.

After two days of intense cleaning, you can back off and continue to take a lower dose and continue to cleanse at a slower pace.

You can get Oxy-Powder on the internet.

Second day of the colon cleanse and fast

During the second day you can drink different kinds of juice and eat 2-6 apples. You can drink any kind of juice be it fruit or vegetable. A combination of fruit and vegetable juice is good.

The juices to drink are listed below in the section called, "Foods You Should Be Eating"

Third day of the colon cleanse and fast

The third day is like the second day where you can drink different kinds of juice and eat 2-6 apples. You can drink any kind of juice be it fruit or vegetable. A combination of fruit and vegetable juice is good

Fourth Day, after the fast is done

After you have finished your three-day fast, start eating soft foods to gently adjust your system to food. Here are some of the foods you can eat during the fourth day out of your fast,

- Baked potato
- Fruit salad
- Fruit smoothie
- Light soup
- Oatmeal, multigrain cereal
- Salad
- Natural Yogurt

You can prepare a fruit smoothie as listed in the last chapter of this e-book. Each morning I prepare a strawberry, or whatever is in season, smoothie and add up to 4 special nutrients to power it up.

9: Step 4 - Essential Fatty Acids And Acne

Getting sufficient essential fatty acids is of prime importance in clearing acne. It's these fatty acids that help to control the production of androgens – the hormones that surge during your teenage years. These androgens, which causes excess sebum oil, clog skin follicle and contribute to creating your acne.

The three fatty acids you need to get daily are omega-3, omega-6, and omega-9. You need more omega 3, fish oil, than omega 6. Actually, you need to balance your omega 3 with your omega 6.

When you are deficient in the essential fatty acids, you will have,

- a weaken immune system
- inflammatory disorders
- poor skin
- skin eruptions and other wounds that won't heal
- sebum production increase (this is what happens when you have acne)
- sebaceous glands size increase.

Eating essential oils is necessary to provide the right oils that are used in the sebaceous glands. These oils can come from straight vegetable oils or from oils in specific foods such as nuts and seeds.

Use flax seed oil (omega-3 oil) and olive oil (omega-6 oil) in your salads. These are the best oils to eat and are called polyunsaturated fatty acids. The other oil that is even better for you is called monounsaturated fatty acid, omega-9. This oil is found in avocados and in other oils, but in small quantities.

Most diets people have contain an excess of omega-6 oil, so mostly likely you need to concentrate on getting more omega-3 oil into your diet.

You can get omega-3 oil from,

- avocados
- sesame seeds
- pumpkin seeds
- walnuts
- dark leafy green vegetables (spinach, mustard greens, kale)
- wheat germ oil
- salmon
- sardines
- albacore tuna

Or, you can take one to two tablespoon of flax seed oil, omega-3 oil, each day. This will give you the amount of omega-3 oil that your body needs. You can add this oil to your morning cereal, soups, smoothies, salads and other liquid foods.

You can get omega-6 oil from,

- Flaxseed oil
- Flaxseeds
- grape seed oil
- pistachio nuts
- olives
- olive oil
- sunflower seeds
- chicken
- evening primrose oil
- pumpkin seeds

- pine nuts

Taking 2-3 tablespoons of omega-6 oil a day will give you the amount of this oil that your body needs. You can add olive oil and other oils into your salad with the flax seed oil.

You can get omega-9 oil from,

- Olive oil
- Avocados
- Peanuts
- Cashews
- Almonds
- Olives
- sesame oil
- pecans
- pistachio nuts

Taking around 1 ½ tablespoon of olive oil per day will give you the omega-9 oil that your body needs.

Other oils that are good for the skin are,

- Apricot kernel oil
- Coconut oil
- Peanut oil
- Almond oil
- Sesame oil
- Sunflower oil
- Wheat germ oil

Use these oils on salads or add a tablespoon to juice or to a smoothie. Use only olive oil, coconut oil, sesame oil and sunflower oil for cooking. But, minimize the use of these oils in cooking. It is always best to use coconut oil to cook, since this oil can withstand higher temperatures than the other oils before it breaks down. Once oils breaks down due to high temperatures, free radicals are formed which attack your internal tissues.

Fish Oils

In addition to supplying your diet with omega-3 and omega-6 oils, you need to supplement your diet with fish oil. Fish oil contains EPA and DHA fatty acids.

Normally, enzymes in your body break down omega-6 into these fatty acids,

- Dihomo-gamma-linolenic acid (DGLA)
- Arachidonic Acid (AA)
- Eicosapentaenoic Acid (EPA)
- Docosahexaenoic Acid (DHA).

These four fatty acids eventually change into prostaglandins.

What are prostaglandins?

Prostaglandins are chemical hormones that come from omega-3 and omega-6 oils and that help, regulate every function in your cells and organs.
Prostaglandins also keep androgen hormones in control so that excess sebum is not produce in the hair follicle, which results in acne.

This is the reason why Essential Fatty Acids – Omega-3 and Omega-6 – are critical foods to eat or supplement with.

However, eating plenty essential fatty acids may not insure that you produce enough EPA and DHA, which produce the essential prostaglandins.

It is critical for your acne and more importantly for your health that you get enough EPA and DHA in your cells and organs so they can produce the required prostaglandins.

To increase the prostaglandins in your cell walls, it is

necessary for you to take a fish supplement, which contains both the EPA and DHA.

Of course eating salmon, halibut, and mackerel twice a week will be a plus in providing your body with more EPA and DHA.

Here's what to use daily. Spectrum Essentials puts out an excellent product called

- Omega-3 Norwegian Fish Oil
- Two capsules contain
- EPA – 360mg
- DHA – 240mg
- Omega-3 – 892mg
- Stearic, Lauric, Palmitic Acids – 508 mg.

Using the Omega-3 Norwegian Fish Oil is critical in getting relief from acne, so take two capsules per meal and don't forget to add some to your Scotty's face cream.

When your body creates prostaglandins, it creates a good prostaglandin and a bad prostaglandin. Here's how to encourage the production of good prostaglandins.

Maintain a ratio of two times more omega-6 than omega-3 in your diet.

Eating too much omega-6 can lead to producing excess bad prostaglandins.

Take a multi-vitamin and minerals with your meals to provide nutrients for breaking down the essential fatty acids into prostaglandins.

Reduce the amount of meat, saturated fat, dairy, and eggs you eat to reduce the production of AA, which blocks the activities of the good prostaglandins.

Eat cold water fish at least twice a week to provide EPA and DHA to your diet.

Twenty percent of your diet calories should be good fats – omega oils and fish oil. This is essential for controlling the excess activity of your hormones and reducing the inflammation of your acne.

10: Step 5 - Making Changes To Your Diet

Changing your diet will be an important step in keep your facial skin healthy and smooth. Even though many dermatologist and doctors don't see the connection between the food that you eat and acne, it does not mean the food you eat is not important in clearing your acne.

If the doctors were right about food and acne, then they would easily be able to help you clear your acne with their drugs. Drugs can give you temporary relief, if they work at all, but as you use them they can also give you some unpleasant side effects.

In her book, Food And Healing, 1986, Annemarie Colbin, points out,

"In a systems view of the body, input of all kinds relates to output of all kinds. Food, therefore, would have a definite relationship to matter pushed out through the skin. I am continually amazed that dermatologists persist in viewing the skin as merely a protective envelope for the body, ascribing its eruptions to 'viruses' and imprecise malfunctions and supporting the myth that 'diet has nothing to do with acne."

Foods to Avoid Eating

If you smoke, drink alcohol or drink coffee, then this program will not work well for you. When you have these addictions, your body minerals and vitamins will be out of balance and it will be difficult to achieve any state of good health.

So, here are they foods that you need to stop eating. You don't need to stop eating these foods instantly. Not many people can do this. You need to do this gradually. I know it will be hard to stop eating some of these foods that you have enjoyed, over the years, but you have to ask yourself the question,

"Do I want to be acne free or a junk food addict?"

The choice is yours and I know you will make the right decision, so here is the list,

White Bread – This is considered junk food since it is void of any vitality for your body. It is hard to digest and causes constipation

Chocolate – some chocolate is better than others. Those that have saturated fats such milk, butter and sugars are not good for your health and definitely not good for your skin. There is cocoa that is semisweet that is better than milk chocolate found in candy.

Fried Fatty foods – fried foods, butter, chesses, beef

Foods in packages – All foods in packages or boxes are junk food. They are considered dead food and provide no life force to your body. They take from you because they use up minerals, vitamins, and digestive enzymes during digestion. They contain no fiber, so they cause constipation.

Foods with artificial flavors and preservatives – These are non-foods that are super toxic. Your body does not know what to do with them, so it stores them in your body as toxic waste.

Milk, ice cream, hard chesses – these foods cause allergies and cause mucus to form. This mucus coats the colon and other internal surfaces and interferes with the function of that area. Bacteria and other pathogens enjoy living in this mucus film. This mucus also tries to escape through the face when you have too much of it in the body. If you cannot digest dairy products, this can cause you to have acne.

Sodas are the worst drink you can take. They contain plenty of sugar and phosphoric acid.

Sugar is considered a white poison. It creates so many health problems in the body that the FDA should outlaw it.

Salt – avoid salt only because it has iodine. Iodine has been shown to cause acne. However, salt has sodium and this mineral forces your body to retain water.

Excess Vitamin B12 – can aggravate or produce acne

Sugar

Sugar is the first thing you should pullout of your diet immediately. Eating sugar is responsible for so many serious diseases. It is considered a poison by good health professionals and comes in many dinguses. Here are some forms,

White sugar (sucrose, brown sugar maple syrup, molasses)

- Fructose
- Glucose
- Maltose
- Lactose
- Corn syrup
- Honey

Eating or drinking any artificial sweetener is even more deadly. The dangers in using these sweeteners are totally underestimated. The liver sees them as a poison.

Eating excess sugar leads to diabetes. This means your pancreas is being over worked and cannot release enough insulin to use the sugar in your blood. A compromised pancreas has a reduced output of digestive enzymes, which leads to undigested food in your colon. This undigested food causes colon toxins that eventually get into your blood stream.

Most all foods in cans, packages, bags, boxes, or cartons have sugar in some form. Read the labels and buy only those foods that have less sugar or no sugar.

Foods You Should Be Eating

- Fruit juices
- Fruits
- Vegetable juices
- Vegetables
- Grains
- Seed and nuts
- Good Oils
- Protein
- Water

Fruit Juices To Drink

Drinking fruit juices helps to bring vitamins and minerals quickly into your blood, where they can go to the skin and supply what is necessary for healthy skin. Minerals quickly neutralize skin acids and bring the skin's pH back to normal – slightly acidic.

Juices have antibacterial action and contain digestive enzymes that help you to digest protein and fat.

Because of the vitamins, minerals, digestive enzymes, pure water, and nutrients that juices have, they have the power to cleanse your body of toxic wastes.

Here are some juices to drink.

Apple juice

Drink at least 2 glasses of this juice every day. Apple juice has a high level of minerals and vitamins, which makes it ideal for skin health.

Apricot – berry juice

Mix equal parts of apricot and berry juice and add a little honey to taste. Drink one cup in the morning. Place the other two glasses into a thermos and drink one more glass at noon and one at dinner.

Cherry juice

Cherry juice is a powerful drink. Because it has so many minerals, it will make your body more alkaline. It neutralizes acid waste in your blood, lymph liquid, and wherever it goes. It will also help in keeping you regular.

Lemon Juice

Lemon juice is one of the best juices you can drink for your skin health. It contains many minerals, which will eliminate acid waste. Lemon juice will help constipation, liver disorders, reduce mucus accumulation, improve digestion, reduce infections, and help to clear skin disorders.

One way I use lemon juice is to squeeze the juice of one lemon into 8 or so ounces water and drink it first thing in the morning. You can also carry unsweetened lemon water in a thermos and drink it during the day.

Melons

Melon juice is also an excellent drink for acne. It is almost a perfect food in that it has many vitamins and minerals. It is most helpful with constipation and kidney and skin disorders.

Orange and grapefruit

Prepare half and half of orange and grapefruit juice using a hand juicer. The flavor is extremely tasty. The combination of these two fresh fruits will give you a powerful start in the morning. They will give you a vitamin C boost, with plenty of flavonoids and minerals.

These combined fruits will cleanse your intestinal tract, help in blood disorders, liver disorders, lung disorders, and skin infections.

Orange and lemon juice

Mix 3 parts of orange juice with one part lemon juice. Add a little water and honey and put into a thermos. Drink the juice all day long for glowing skin.

Lemon juice helps the skin to rejuvenate and grow new skin. It helps the skin to flake off old skin and improve the skin's metabolism.

Other juices to drink

There are many other fruit juices to drink. Here are a few more.

- Peach juice
- Pear juice
- Pineapple juice
- Prune juice
- Strawberry juice

Try to use organic fruits when making your juice. It is better to make your own juices since most bottled juice contain no life force or natural live enzymes. Drink the juices soon after you juice them. If you want, put them in a thermos for later in the day.

Fruits

Eating fruits that are red or orange in color will help improve your skin health. Here are the fruits you should be eating.

Apples – eat 2 – 3 apples a day while clearing your acne. Apples are good for skin health. Eat at least two a day. Eat organic apples, because you can eat the skins and most pectin is in the skin, which helps with constipation. Apples contain ascorbic acid, bioflavonoids, fiber, pectin, quercetin, minerals, and vitamins.

Apricots – eat as many as you like. Apricots are a high source of minerals, fiber, and beta-carotene and will help control acne. (A precursor to vitamin A) They help to relieve or prevent constipation.

Bananas – eat only one banana a day. Bananas have the phytochemicals fructoOligosaccharides, which feeds the good bacterial in your colon. By feeding the good bacteria, you prevent the bad bacteria from overtaking the colon and producing toxic acids that get to the skin.

Blackberries – help cleanse the blood and are good for constipation. They help a weak kidney and are good for creating good skin on your face.

Blueberries – are a good blood cleanser. They are also good for constipation and various skin disorders.

Cantaloupes – are high in vitamin A, C and have many other minerals. This makes it good for any type of skin problems

Cherries – are good blood cleansers and help the liver, kidney. They promote regular bowel movements.

Figs – are high in fiber and help to reduce constipation.

Grapefruits – helps to dissolve and eliminate poisons from drugs and improving the liver function.

Grapes – help cleanse the body, build blood, and build the body. It is good for constipation, skin, and liver disorders.

Mango – is good for kidney inflammation. It contains a lot of minerals, which help to neutralize acid waste.

Strawberries – have been shown to have strong anti-acne activity. They are high in pectin content, which helps to keep your bowels moving.

Pineapples – contains many vitamins and minerals. It contains Papain, which helps to digest protein. They are useful in excess mucus, digestive problems, intestinal worms, and constipation.

These fruits below are useful for acne, since they have an antibiotic effect,

- Grapes
- Plums
- Figs
- Raspberries
- Blueberries
- Honey
- Apple juice
- Grape juice
- Orange juice

Vegetable juices

Vegetable juices are absorbed quickly into your bloodstream. As a result, your cells are quickly provided with nutrients that feed them and that wash away waste. Vegetable juices give you the opportunity to get quick relief from various body conditions such as acne and constipation.

Eating and drinking vegetables provide you with minerals and nutrients that build your blood, tissue, bones, and cells.

It is minerals that build every part of your body. It is minerals that keep your body's pH at the required level. It is minerals that keep your body alkaline, by neutralizing body acids.

Concentrate on putting minerals into your body by eating and drinking plenty of fruits and vegetables.

Carrot apple juice

Drink carrot juice every day. You can mix carrot juice with apple juice to create a better juice.

Carrot juice contains many vitamins and minerals. It is high in beta-carotene. Carrot juice will enhance your skin health and help you eliminate acne.

Carrot, spinach, and apple juice

A combination of carrot, spinach and apple juice is a powerful drink for cleaning the colon, relieving constipation and improving your skin conditions.

To make this drink, juice 3-4 carrots and a bunch of spinach. Then add juiced apples to make this drink more drinkable.

Whole Vegetables

Phytochemicals are all of the chemicals that exist in vegetables and fruits. There are so many phytochemicals that scientists have yet to investigate and learn about all of them.

Here are the vegetables that you should be eating the most of, so you can support the cleansing of your face and eliminating acne.

Carrots – contain a rich source of vitamin A-like carotenoids. These phytochemicals have been shown to enhance the health of skin and repair it, when it is damaged.

Cabbage – helps to detoxify the body of harmful chemicals from air and food additives.

Celery – helps to reduce nervous tension. It contains many the mineral sodium that helps to neutralize body acid waste and is high in fiber.

Cucumber – helps to reduce acne problems because it is high in silicon and sulfur. It is also a diuretic, which helps flow more water through the kidney to clean out your blood.

Broccoli – is rich in beta carotene, a precursor to vitamin A, which is good for the skin.

Garlic – is a natural antibiotic and will help relieve skin bacterial infections. Use garlic in all of your cooking.

Green pepper – The nutrients in green peppers are good for liver health and constipation. Its minerals are good for neutralizing acid waste. It's a good source of vitamin C.

Radishes – help to digest your food. Good digestion is necessary to avoid constipation and to keep the liver and pancreas strong.

Sprouts – provide plenty of vitamins and minerals, which help to reduce body acids.

Watercress – helps to prevent vitamin and mineral deficiencies at the skin surface. It provides Vitamin A, B1, B2, C, iron, manganese, copper, and calcium.

Grains

Brown rice – contain many amino acids that help rebuild skin tissue.

Whole grains – these grains contain vitamin B and an array of minerals.

Oats – use them in the morning with honey, bananas, or raisins. Oats have an anti-inflammatory effect on the skin and help to keep you regular.

Seeds and nuts

Almonds - Almonds contain protein, the B vitamins, calcium, iron, potassium, magnesium, and phosphorus. Use them as a snack. These small nuts help to build muscles and tissue. This is the best nut to eat.

Flax seeds – These seeds are known for containing plenty of omega 3 oil, an essential oil for life. The also contain fiber when used ground up and put into smoothies. Omega 3 is also an anti-inflammatory oil, which is good for acne.

Pecans – This is a good nut to eat. It contains Vitamin A, B's, C, calcium, iron, phosphorus, and potassium. Use them as snacks.

Pine nuts – These nuts also one of the best to eat. They contain vitamin A, C, B's, protein and iron.

Sesame seeds – They are high in calcium, phosphorus, and potassium. They are helpful in relieving various skin diseases, such as acne by reducing the swelling. Spread them on your salads or put them into your smoothies.

Sunflower seeds – These seeds should be used as a snack. They are high in protein, calcium and vitamin A. They provide nutrients for building the whole body and are good for dry skin.

All of these nuts and seeds should be eaten raw. Use them between meals as snacks and not right after a meal. Heating and other processing will kill the life force of nuts or seeds and reduce the quality of the vitamins and minerals they have.

Protein

Eating excess meat is harmful to your health. Eating too much meat, more than 2-4 ounces per day, has been found to contribute to narrowing of the arteries.

If you do physical labor and are involved in a lot of movement in your work, then you should eat more protein than 2-4 ounces per day. Just make sure that the meat has a minimum of additives and preservatives.

Remember, meat is high in saturated fat, which blocks the activity of EPA and DHA, which controls the activity of your hormones.

Meat and bread is a big contributor to creating constipation. Meat is difficult to digest and many times it will get into the colon partial digested. This condition benefits the bad bacteria and allows them to dominate the colon and create constipation.

Because meat and bread have little fiber, they move slowly in the colon, which leads to constipation and eventually to some type of colon inflammation or hemorrhoids. For this reason, you should always eat a salad when you eat meat or bread.

Bad bacteria, decaying meat and other undigested food contribute to the build up of toxic matter in the colon. This is the type of condition you should try to avoid, if you have acne. You need the fecal matter in your colon to move daily out the rectum; otherwise, toxic matter will build up and end up in your blood stream.

11: Step 6 - Eating Breakfast Using Body Cycles

Natural Body Cycles

Here's some information that will help you achieve even more results in your efforts to get rid of acne. It is call "Using the Natural Body Cycles" for achieving maximum health.

By learning how to assist your "Natural Body Cycles", you will be in tune with what your body is doing to maintain your health.

Getting in tune with your Natural Body Cycles requires changes in the way you eat. Since all of us are addicted to the way we eat, it is, sometimes, difficult to change these habits.

Using this method to gain better health, you may experience some side effects, because you will be eliminating more body toxins and body wastes. The side effects may be headaches, stomach upsets, body pains, or similar types of symptoms. These conditions will not last and will disappear as you get rid of more toxins. So if you experience these side effects, don't let them stop you from moving forward on this eating pattern.

Your body has 3 natural body cycles. Here you will learn only about body cycle 1. This cycle occurs from 4am to 12 noon. During this cycle, your body is in the elimination process. It is this time your body is eliminating waste from your body in the form of sweating, urine, and bowel movements.

You can assist your body in eliminating wastes by drinking fruit juices, tea, special drinks and eating fruits and vegetables when you first wake up to noon time. Here is what you can do.

Morning Breakfast Drinks

First, drink one glass of water with half the juice of one lemon.

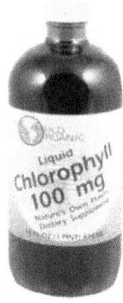

30 minutes later drink a green drink in one of two ways. You can put 1 to 2 tablespoons of liquid chlorophyll in 8 oz. of water or a capful of your favorite green powder in 8 oz. of water.

For the <u>chlorophyll drink</u>, add the juice of 1/2 lemon juice to give it some flavor. For the <u>green power</u> drinks add some honey so it is easier to drink.

Or, you can you make a tea of ginger and green tea and drink this. To do this, buy some green tea bags and fresh ginger. Boil both cut up ginger and a green tea bag. Add some honey to give it a sweet taste.

After Your Morning Drink

After you finish your morning drink wait about 1/2 hour before you start your breakfast. Eat only fruits for breakfast. Choose from any of these fruit preparations and choose different ones to eat on different days.

Eating fruits and drinking only juices from morning to noon is part of the body cycle I process. It's in the morning that you help your body to eliminate body toxins that have accumulated during the night. Since fruits and juices have a short digestion cycle, this cycle helps you to better eliminate waste from your body every morning.

Here are a few morning breakfast suggestions:

1. Cut and prepare a bowl of various fresh fruits. Do not add any toppings.

2. Cut and mix watermelon and cantaloupe slices together. Do not mix this fruit with other types of fruit.

3. Prepare a fruit pudding in a blender using 3 or 4 different fruits listed in the previous chapter. This is a great way to get plenty of nutrients into your body fast. It also fills and satisfies your hunger. Use different fruits or use the same ones for a few days. You can add a touch of honey, lecithin, or different juices to adjust the consistency of the pudding.

   If you have flax seeds or any other seeds that you like, use a coffee grinder to grind a tablespoon or so, and then add this to your pudding
   You can prepare a mango, pineapple, strawberry, banana, apple, peach, and apricot pudding. Just experiment with the different fruit puddings you can prepare.

   You can put some of this pudding in a thermos and use it for snacks during the morning or afternoon break.

4. Prepare a smoothie as shown in the smoothie chapter. Drink part of it for breakfast and the rest for your breaks.

5. On occasion you can eat a pouched egg or a small amount of whole oats, but not the quick cooking oats. You can use apple juice to dilute the oats and add a banana and raisins. You can do this once a week, if you like.

Fruit Pudding

Next mix a fruit pudding to take to work for a snack. Here are two different things you can do with a blender. Take these blended fruits to work in a thermos to eat when you get there.

Put into a blender

Two small or one large banana
One mango
Pineapple
One apple
1/4 of a papaya (if available)
Small amount of apple juice to make this blend into a pudding

Blend all of this for 1 – 2 minutes.

You can add lecithin granules or powdered vitamin C to make it more a tart and to preserve it.

Pineapple Smoothie

Mix the following in a blender to create a smoothie.

1-2 cups of fresh pineapples
1/2 cups apple slices
1/4 cup fresh apple juice
1/4 cup rice dream (more or less as needed)
1 small banana
1-teaspoon lecithin
1-teaspoon flax seed oil (use grounded seeds)
2 teaspoons bran (oat or rice)
1/2 of plain yogurt

You can choose different fruits to create new smoothies.

You can alternate using the pudding and smoothie. Also you can change the fruit from pineapples to mango or strawberries. Don't use a smoothie every day. Use the smoothie to break the monotony of eating only sliced fruits.

Now, about 1/2 hour or so before lunch, eat your last fruit.

Morning Snack time

During your morning and afternoon break, it's time to open your thermos and have a good snack. Make sure you take your snack break. Use only fruits, vegetables, nuts, and vegetable soups for your snacks. These types of snacks help you to digest your food better and also activate peristaltic colon action. They give you fiber and many of the minerals you need to make your body more alkaline and to improve your skin.

To make your body more alkaline, use fresh fruits such as grapes, apples, watermelon, cantaloupes, apricots, peaches, pineapples, strawberries, other berries, mangos, and so on.

Use drinks like apple, cherry, prune, pineapple, tomato, carrot, and so on.

There you have it, the breakfast. This should become your new eating habit. You will find that eating in this way you will not be hungry until your lunch.

Fruit and Fiber

Here is a list of fruits that give you the most fiber. Try to get up to 30 to 35 grams of fiber every day. If you are short on fiber for the day look at this list of fruits and eat the ones that give you more fiber. Also notice the fruit serving and if you want more fiber double the serving.

FRUIT LIST	Fruit Serving	Fiber
Apple, unpeeled, small	1 (4 oz.)	4
Applesauce, unsweetened	½ cup	1
Apples, dried	4 rings	2
Apricots, fresh	4 whole	1
Apricots, dried	8 halves	4
Apricots, canned	½ cup	1
Banana, small	1 (4 oz.)	1
Blackberries	¾ cup	5
Blueberries	¾ cup	5
Cantaloupe, small	1 cup cubes	2
Cherries, fresh	12	2

Cherries, sweet, canned	½ cup	1
Dates	3	2-3
Figs, dried	2	2
Fruit cocktail	½ cup	1
Grapefruit, large	½	1
Grapes	17	1
Honeydew melon	1 slice	1
Kiwi	1	3
Mandarin oranges, canned	¾ cup	1
Mango, small	½ cup	1
Nectarine, small	1	2
Orange, small	1 (6 ½ oz.)	3
Papaya	½ fruit	3 Peach,
fresh	1	2
Peaches, canned	½ cup	1
Pear, large, fresh	½ (4 oz.)	4
Pears, canned	½ cup	1
Pineapple, fresh	¾ cup	1
Pineapple, canned	½ cup	1
Plums, small	2	2
Raisins	2 tbsp.	1
Raspberries	1 cup	8
Strawberries	1 ¼ cup	4
Tangerines, small	2	2
Watermelon	1 ¼ cup	1

12: Step 7 & 8 - Vitamins & Minerals That Reduce Acne

Vitamins

Here are some of the vitamins and minerals you should be taking to help you get rid of acne.

- B6, 25 – 150 mg in a B vitamin complex
- B5 pantothenic acid, 500 – 1000 mg per day
- Vitamin A (water soluble), 25,000 to 40,000 IU – take just before meals. Taking more than 50,000 IU requires a Doctors approval
- Vitamin C, buffered, 1000mg three time a day
- Vitamin E, 400 IU two times a day before meals for a total of 800 IU a day.

A word of caution: Do not take more than 50, 000 IU unit of vitamin A since it can be toxic at higher levels. If you experience any symptoms with 50,000 IU's of vitamin A, then you should back off to 25,000 units.

Minerals

Here are some of the minerals you should be taking to help control and eliminate acne.

Calcium Hydroxyapatite Complex a tablet after each meal. Take the quantity listed on the label.

Chromium 200 – 500 ugm or micrograms a day

Mineral electrolytes

Zinc gluconate 25 – 60 mg a day (zinc is one of the most important nutrient to add to your diet) Zinc works to reduce the male sex hormone dihyrdrotestosterone (DHT), which in excess will produce acne. Do not take over 100 mg unless you consult with a Doctor.

Word of Caution: After you have gain relief from acne, you can discontinue the use of the above supplements and get back to your normal supplementation program. Continual use of high doses of vitamins and minerals will offset your natural body's chemical balance and is detrimental to your health in the long run.

13: Step 9 - Special Acne Supplements

There are seven special supplements that you should consider taking to improve your overall health for now and for the future. These supplements will improve your immune system and help to clear and prevent future acne.

Look at these supplements and take the one that you feel will give you the most benefits for your health.

- Oxygen Elements Plus
- Electrolyte Minerals
- Systemic Enzymes
- Digestive enzymes
- Flax Seed Oil
- Lecithin
- Chlorophyll and Lemon
- Oxygen Elements Plus

The skin needs plenty of oxygen to keep it clean and free of bacteria. Using a product like Oxygen Elements Plus gives you at least 10-20% more oxygen in your blood. Oxygen Plus can be obtained on the internet.

Increasing the oxygen in your blood is now a necessity for normal health. Your body needs more oxygen than you presently get from the air you breathe, so that your body functions normally.

With the present oxygen in the air, you are providing a body host for all kinds of bacteria, parasites, and virus, which like a low oxygen environment.

The amount of oxygen you have in your body that is available to your cells is dependent on conditions such as,

- Acid in the body
- Excess Nonfood waste products in the body
- Pathogens in the body

These three items, acid, nonfoods, and pathogens use up your oxygen. The oxygen that is left over is then used for your body's needs. So the more you have of these three items, the less oxygen you will have to supply your body's needs. Drinking Chlorophyll liquid in the morning gives you more oxygen.

Electrolyte Minerals

The skin needs plenty of minerals. You can use a mineral supplement to get this and here is a list of some of the best products to use.

Alkalife – this is a liquid that contains ionic sodium and potassium. By adding 2 drops in a glass of distilled water, the water pH is changed from 7.0 to 8.0. This change makes the water alkaline and is the type of water you want to be drinking to give you more minerals to neutralize acids.

Crystalloid Electrolytes – This is the form of minerals that are in your lymph liquid surrounding your cells. These ionic minerals are similar to the electrolytes that keep your car battery charged. Without ionic minerals in your body, your body will lose its life energy. The more minerals you have in your body, the more life force you will have.

Systemic Enzymes

If you have scars or pockmarks that have recently occurred from acne, you may be able to clear them by using a product called Vitalzym. Check Google for Vitalzym.

You're not going to hear this from your doctor or

dermatologist, but systemic enzymes, such as serapeptase, can remove excess fibrin, which makes up scar tissue.

Systemic enzymes have a different function from digestive enzymes. Systemic enzymes work in the body organs, tissue, skin, and joints to remove excess fibrin, which accumulates in these areas. Systemic enzymes,

- Bring nutrient to damaged area
- Enhance wellness
- Help to speed repair of damage tissue
- Improves blood and lymphatic circulation
- Reduce inflammation
- Remove waste products
- Stimulate immune system

Digestive Enzymes

Digestive enzymes are used to help you digest food that you eat. If you eat mostly processed foods, these foods don't have digestive enzymes to help digest themselves, so your body has to pull them from deep in the body to do digestion in the stomach or intestines.

Over many years of eating processed food instead of live food, like raw fruits and vegetables, your digestive enzyme supply will diminish and you will not digest food as good as when you were younger.
Supplementing your diet with digestive enzymes and taking them with every meal will insure that you digest your food properly.

This will reduce the amount of undigested food that gets into your colon where toxic matter is formed.

Flax seed oil

Flax seed oil has an anti-inflammatory effect on the body and on skin diseases. It will help to reduce or relieve the inflammation of your acne. Take one teaspoon to one table spoon a day.

Lecithin

Lecithin is made from soybeans and is found in health food stores in yellow granules. It is an emulsifier, which is a substance that helps fats and nonfat to mixed and stay together without separating.

In the blood it keeps the fats from forming large globes, which can create problems, if your arteries are narrow. Lecithin also has many other benefits such as,

- Improves digestion and absorption of essential fatty acids
- Improves skin problems
- Improves memory
- Lowers cholesterol

Add 1-2 tablespoons of granules to your smoothies. Add one or two teaspoons to your soups or other liquid food. Sprinkle one teaspoon on your fresh salads.

Chlorophyll and lemon

Here is one of the best drinks you can take. It's a drink that combines liquid chlorophyll and one lemon juice. This drink helps to build your blood and bring more oxygen to your cells. If you don't eat a lot of greens, chlorophyll can help to provide the chlorophyll that greens provide.

Why You Should Take This drink

Chlorophyll is one of the best ways to detoxify the colon fast. It also helps the skin to keep healthy by acting as an

- antioxidant

- anti-inflammatory
- anti-microbial agent
- absorber of heavy metals in the colon

Here are some of the benefits you will get from drinking chlorophyll,

- Heals open wounds inside your body
- Increases re-growth of tissues
- Helps to heal sores in your mouth
- Acts as a antiseptic
- Destroys bacteria
- Brings more oxygen to your cells
- Give protection from low levels of radiation such as TV, computers, microwaves, and hospital equipment
- Reduces toxins in the colon and body
- Helps to purify the liver
- Helps sores heal faster
- Reduces pain from inflammation

Here's how to prepare it first thing in the morning,

- Place 2-3 tablespoon of plain liquid chlorophyll in an 8 oz glass
- Squeeze the juice of one whole lemon into the glass
- Fill the glass with 8 oz. of water
-

By adding one lemon to this drink, you give this drink some flavor. You may try adding chlorophyll to some other juice, if you like. Other juices work just as well.

You cannot overdose on chlorophyll liquid, so you can drink 2 ounces plus the juice of one lemon in an 8 oz. glass of water.

14: Step 10 - Herbal Mixtures That Help Clear Acne

Using herbal mixtures can sometimes increase the acne activity temporarily. Do not panic, since herbs are a powerful way to cleanse the blood and start the acne healing process.

Mix a tea, which contains the following herbs,

- Figwort 1 ounce
- Turkey corn 1 ounce
- Echinacea 1 ounce
- Thuja 1 ounce
- Yellow dock 1 ounce
- Arctium lappa ½ ounce
- Iris versicolor ½ ounce

You can also make a tea using any one of the following teas. Just pick 2 to 3 of the herbs and make a tea. Sometimes the tea may need some flavoring, so add some honey. Drink the tea throughout the day.

- Burdock
- Dandelion
- Echinacea
- Fragrant valerian
- Goldenseal
- Ivy
- Marshmallow root
- Purslane
- Watercress
- Wild strawberry leaves
- Yarrow root

You can sometimes find a box of premixed herbal teas that are for acne at your favorite health food store.

Herbal Extract

Here's an herbal extract that is designed for acne. Its main function is to improve the liver function, purify the blood, reduce acne inflammation, and fight acne bacterial infections.

This herbal extract is a liquid and is taken in water or as drops into your mouth.

The name of the herbal extract is Burdock-Sarsaparilla Compound and contains the following herbs:

Burdock mature seed - helps to purify the liver, balance hormones, neutralizes acid, anti-inflammatory, and useful in purifying the blood.

Jamaican sarsaparilla root – helps scaling skin, blood purifying, reduces itching, and helps balance hormones.

Nettle mature seed – is anti-inflammatory for the skin, neutralizes acid waste with its high mineral content.

Yellow dock root – rich in iron and works to improve liver function, helps build good blood, helps to purify blood and lymphatic liquid, and helps increase bile, which helps to reduce constipation.

Spilanthes flowing herb – improves immunity to fight bacterial infections on the skin.

Sassafras root bark – blood cleansing, anti-inflammatory for the skin.

This is excellent herbal remedy and is not very expensive. If you can find it at a health food store, it should cost around $10.00. If not, then you can order it on the Internet and pay around $16.00, shipping included.

Here's how to take this herbal extract.

Take 30 – 35 drops in water three times a day. Take it for on 6 days, then let your body rest and start again after the seventh day.

A word of caution: Do not use this remedy as the only method to get rid of acne. This has to be used in combination with the 12 steps outlined in this program.

Foot Spa

In the book by William L. Fischer called Hidden Secrets of Super Perfect Health at Any Age, Book II, 1986, chapter 10, The F-M Circulizer System is revealed. Fischer discusses the use of an herbal footbath. A footbath can be used to bring herb nutrients into your body.

This book was written in 1986 and Fischer claims this herbal footbath has been in use overseas since 1946!

If you already have foot spa, thank your mother, sister, or whoever bought it for you, because you're in for a treat. If you don't have one, then with $20 or $30 you can get one.

When you use a heated footbath, veins in your feet start to expand. Over a period of 15-20 minute, the warm water affects your entire vascular (blood) system and you get improved blood circulation.

By adding herbs to the hot water, minerals and other phytochemicals from the herbs enter the soles of your feet and into your blood stream.

This means that you can introduce herbal phytochemicals into your blood stream using the footbath. During your footbath, these herbal chemicals quickly circulated throughout your body and get to work neutralizing acid, killing bacteria, and improving your skin circulation.

Here are the herbs you need to use for your skin and how to prepare and use an herbal footbath.

This herbal combination was taken and modified slightly from a book written by Daniel B. Mowrey, Ph.D., called The Scientific Validation of Herbal Medicine, 1986. In his book Mowrey says,

"This (herbal) blend attacks external skin disorders from within, purifying the blood, carrying away waste, reinforcing the blood's ability to ward off infectious agents."

The herbal combination to use is,

Dandelion root – purifies blood and improves liver function

Yellow dock root – purifies blood, helps liver, is anti-bacterial

Saraparilla root – has antibiotic action, promotes waste elimination through urine and sweating.

Echinacea – increases immunity and promotes skin healing

Licorice – protects the liver so that it can detoxify the blood better

Kelp – provide minerals and vitamins and binds heavy metal that are bad for health

Chaparral – is anti-microbial making it effective against acne.

Buy one ounce of each herb and mix them. If you can't find one specific herb, use the herbs that you can find.

Here's how to do the herbal footbath,

- Mix all the herbs in a mason jar
- Place 2 tablespoons of herbal mix into 1 ½ cups of water
- Boil the water with herbs – use a glass, porcelain, or stainless steel container
- After the water starts to boil, pull the container of the stove
- Let the tea sit for 15-30 minutes. The longer the tea sits the stronger the tea and its effects
- Prepare your foot spa with water
- Strain the tea to remove leaves and roots
- Poor tea into foot spa
- Place your feet in hot water as high as you can stand for 15 – 30 minutes.

Do your foot spa until you see result in your acne. You can use it every day, every other day or whatever frequency you want. You can also use some of the other herbs I have listed in previous chapters.

15: Step 11 - Brushing Skin to Eliminate Toxins

Brushing your skin while dry and just before taking a shower is a way to stimulate the flow of liquid through lymphatic system and increase the circulating of blood.

Brushing your skin also does the following:

- Removes dry dead cells that can clog your skin

- Opens pores which allow you to excrete more toxins safely

- Activates the nerves near the top of your skin, making your skin work better

- Stimulates the tiny blood vessels near your skin and brings more nutrients and acid neutralizing minerals to your skin.

- Improves your overall health since the skin must eliminate close to 2 pounds of waste through the pores.

If you practice dry brushing your skin, you will see improved beauty and health in your skin.

You can also scrub your skin during your shower and this is an excellent way to do it.

There are two different types of brushes that are designed for dry skin brushing.

- A natural bristle brush

- Loofah with a long handle

When you start bushing for the first time, do it softly and gentle, until your skin gets use to the rough feeling.

If you have not been brushing and scrubbing your skin, then you need to do this only after you have completed the above steps 1 – 5 of the twelve step process.

Because skin brushing promotes release of toxins through the skin, you want to make sure you are not constipated; otherwise you will start to release too many toxins through the skin.

A word of caution: Brush only once a day and do not brush too hard. Excessive brushing over stimulates the skin and can produce unwanted side effects.

But, here is how to dry brush your skin before you take a shower,

Start with gentle light touch circular motions at your face. If you have severe acne, do this gently massage with a clean hot face towel and do not brush your face.

You should always brush only in the direction of your heart. From the feet upward, brush up toward your heart. At the neck, brush downward toward your heart.

After you finishing brushing, about 5 minutes, take a shower to remove the dead and old skin. You may only want to brush your skin during your shower with Loofah.

In the shower, use the Loofa with soap and brush your skin as described above. It is a gentler way to brush your skin and you wash away the skin derby at the same time.

16: Step 12 - Change Your Attitude

There is no way that you can rid yourself of acne without thinking about why you have acne. If you skip this step, you lose an opportunity to connect deeper with your self (mind), which later in life will give you various advantages as you face new life issues.

So, start by being more accepting of yourself. No matter how much you put yourself down or how critical you are of yourself, it will not change the world around you. The world and you are still the same.

So, just get over it. Stop fighting who you are.

Accept yourself as you are and get on with the purpose of your life. Just get on with it. Don't worry about what other people are thinking and doing. That's their problem not yours.

You need to learn how to "face yourself." Is it when you have acne that you don't want to look at yourself and "face who you are?"

If you have acne, there is always some underlying emotions and feelings that are being expressed by your acne. Look into yourself and try to see what you are saying with your acne.

If you cannot find it, see if you can relate it to constipation. Constipation and a toxic colon is typically the cause of acne. But to go one-step further, all physical illness is created by some emotional unbalance that you are holding onto.

Acne is a representation of repressed traumas that you have experienced as a child. Acne can be an expression of those traumas trying to burst out. Your body has a defense mechanism that holds back and buries past traumas.

Some effort has to be make to connect and release these traumas, otherwise as you clear your face these traumas can move to some other parts of your body where they will be unseen and destroy tissue and body functions.

All past suppressed trauma that you have experienced has a representation in the body, internally or externally. This representation can be an internal body weakness or disease. Or it can be topical condition like acne, boils, rashes, eczema, or psoriasis.

Your body protects you from early trauma that could have overwhelmed you, causing death or mental breakdown. It does this by suppressing the pain associated with the trauma. But this suppressed pain needs to be expressed by your body through distortions in your health or appearance.

Good Luck To You

Follow the 12 steps and you will get results. Follow the steps and your face will clear and become smooth and lovable.

17: How To Use The 12 Acne Steps

Thank you for reading and applying this information. This information is for your education and you assume any risk in applying this information. Study it closely and you decide how you want to use it to cure your acne.

Go carefully and test each cream, gel, oil, herb, or other product on a small spot on your skin to look for allergies or major irritations. Stop and dilute the cream or gel, if you get an unpleasant reaction.

You should use both the topical cream process and the twelve steps to help you eliminate acne.

Acne can be a difficult condition to eliminate. But if you are consistent in applying the processes outline here, you will succeed.

You do not have to do each step. But the more steps you do, the better health you will have. Eliminating acne is about improving your eating habits and lifestyle. It's about cleansing your internal organs, so that they function like they should. It's about getting your body back in balance and back to normal.

Once you have eliminated acne or have it under control, you can lessen the supplements that you take. But this should only be done, if you are eating more fruits and vegetables.

Here I outline two programs, giving specifics that you can follow. There are many different 12-step programs you can create with the information I have provided. Here I will give you two that are good and it may not be ones you like. You can adapt a program to the things that don't cost too much or you can buy numerous products to make things easier for you.

But if you are a good experimenter, you can keep your costs down. So let get started.

Low cost program,

Step 1: Keep your face clean – use glycerin or castile soap

Step 2: Use Scotty's acne face cream

Step 3: Relieve constipation - the first day liquid fast - use prune juice and apple juice just one day, the following two days eat apples and drink apple juice or other fruit drinks

Step 4: Make changes to your diet by eliminating some processed foods and adding more raw fruit and vegetables.

Step 5: Drink plenty of distilled water

Step 6: Use the body cycle 1 breakfast

Step 7: Vitamins you should be taking – Vitamin A and a B vitamin complex.

Step 8: Minerals you should be taking – add calcium and zinc.

Step 9: Herbal mixtures to drink or to use – use the Burdock-Sarsaparilla Compound

Step 10: Special supplements to take – take the chlorophyll and lemon juice drink. Use flax seed oil in your salads.

Step 11: Brushing your skin daily

Step 12: Think about what acne is trying to express in your

emotional life. And start making changes in your thought process and start doing things differently.

Higher cost program

Step 1: Keep your face clean – use glycerin or castile soap

Step 2: Use Scotty's acne face cream

Step 3: Relieve constipation with a three day liquid fast - use "Oxy-Powder" the first day and the following days eat apples and drink apple juice or other fruit drinks

Step 4: Making changes to your diet by eliminating some processed foods and adding more raw fruit and vegetables.

Step 5: Drink plenty of distilled water with Alkalife

Step 6: Start using body cycle morning breakfast

Step 7: Take Vitamins – Vitamin A and a B vitamin complex and take additional B5 pantothenic acid, 500 – 1000 mg per day

Step 8: Take Minerals – add calcium, zinc, and Oxygen Elements Plus

Step 9: Herbal mixtures to drink or to use – use the Burdock-Sarsaparilla Compound and do the herbal foot bath.

Step 10: Take special supplement – take chlorophyll and lemon juice drink. Use digestive enzymes. Use flax seed oil in your salad.

Step 11: Brush your skin daily

Step 12: Think about what acne is trying to express in your emotional life. Start changing your thoughts and make changes in your behavior, by being more understanding, flexible, problem solving, and less angry, jealous, and stubborn.

When you have a disagreement with someone, let yourself see what part you had in this disagreement and fix that. Don't always assume it was someone else's fault for what happen. There are always two sides to a problem and you can only fix your side.

18: About The Author And Other Resources

Rudy Silva is a natural consultant nutritionist educated in the United State in Nutrition and Physics. He is a graduate from the San Jose State University in California. He is author of 30 other e-books on natural remedies. He has authored a newsletter in natural remedies for over 4 years. He has many websites promoting special recommended products and information.

Resource page

Here are some of the other kindle e-books about natural remedies that have been written by this author.

Acne Remedies

Natural Help With Acne
Best natural acne treatments: Acne facial

Constipation Remedies

The Best Constipation Remedies
Best Constipated Women Natural Cures
How To Relieve Constipation With Fruits

Essential Fatty Acids

Taking The Mystery Out Of Essential Fatty acids
Amazing Fish Oil Benefits Revealed

Nutrition Remedies

Updated Version - Secret Diet And Nutrition

Secret Healthy Fruit Practices Revealed
Fast Healing Juice Nutrition Therapy: Nutrition Tips 3
Fantastic Alkaline Fruit Benefits Revealed
Calcium (Discover How To Use Calcium To Avoid Devastating Diseases)
Magnesium Nutrition Revealed
Best Nutrition Health Practices
Potassium Health Secrets Revealed
Phosphorus, The Best Brain Food

Stomach Remedies

Acid Reflux: Fast and Easy Cures For Acid Reflux
Asthma Treatment Cures With Remedies
How To Do Natural Colon Cleansing
Gastrointestinal Digestion Secrets Revealed

Misc Remedies

Natural Hair Loss Treatment: Women And Men
Effective Natural Hemorrhoids Treatment
Iron Deficiency Anemia
Secrets To Understanding Behavior
Fast Acting Ear Infection Remedies
Best Impotence Health Diet
What Is A Hiatus Hernia
Best Varicose Vein Treatments?
Make Shampoos At Home Using Natural Ingredients

To see all of the kindle books written by this author, go to this the **Authors Profile Page**.

If you need support or want to promote any of his e-books, please contact him at **rss41@yahoo.com** and expect a reply within 24 hours. He looks forward to hearing from you and is happy to help you understand his material on natural and nutritional health.

Give A Review

And, don't for get to give a review for this e-book at Amazon so that others can gain the benefits of what is in this e-book.

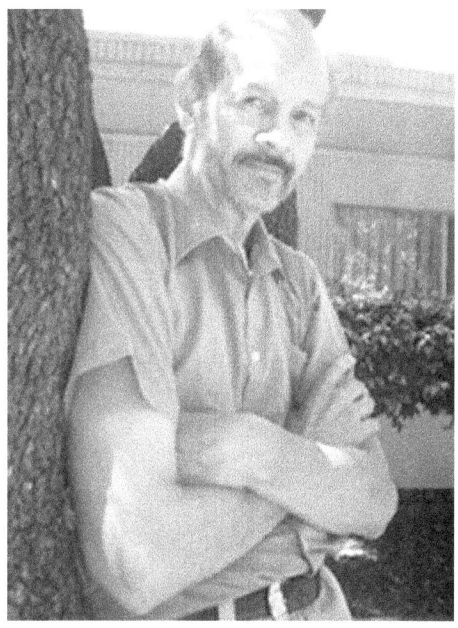

To you, for losing weight, creating better health and more happiness in your life,

Rudy S Silva